How to Navigate
The Medicare Maze

Turning 65 or Otherwise Qualified

Michael J. Kench

A step-by-step guide to help you navigate the complex maze of Medicare, which will teach you the ins-and-outs of the program and help you make sense of its processes.

It will provide timesaving tips to help you avoid common mistakes and any ensuing penalties.

FREE BONUS:
JOIN ME FOR FREE VIDEO TRAINING

Register right now to join me for Free Bonus Video Training. I will be covering Medicare Basics, Medicare Part C, Medicare Part D and Medicare Supplement (Medigap) plans.

Visit http://www.howtonavigatemedicare.com

Table of Contents

Introduction

Welcome to: **How to Navigate the Medicare Maze when You Turn 65 or Qualify for Medicare.**

This step-by-step guide to Medicare will show you how Medicare works as you turn 65 or when you first qualify for Medicare benefits. This book will save you time by breaking down the various parts of Medicare in an easy-to-understand format.

You'll learn what Medicare parts **A, B, C, and D** are, collectively referred to as the "Alphabet Soup" of Medicare. You'll learn what are Medicare Supplement "Medigap" policies (**A–N**) are and what they cover, the differences between **Medicare Advantage** and **Medigap** plans, and why you should consider prescription drug coverage when it first becomes available if your plan does not include one. The book will also show you **how to qualify** for Medicare benefits, **when and how to apply** for coverage, and **how to avoid** any potential **penalty** situations.

At the end of each chapter, you will find a **step-by-step action plan** that will help answer any questions you may have.

Medicare choices and decisions can be overwhelming at times—this book will help guide you and simplify the process by helping you make informed Medicare decisions based on your budget and health care needs.

Chapter 1

What Is Medicare?

Let's look at the Medicare basics. Medicare includes four parts that help you with your health care costs.

Part A, Part B, Part C and Part D.

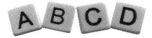

Part A is hospital insurance, which helps pay for in-patient hospital stays in addition to:

- Skilled nursing care
- Home health care
- Hospice care

Part B is medical insurance, which helps pay for:

- Doctor visits
- Medical services and supplies

Parts A and B are known as "Original Medicare."

 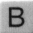

Part C is the Medicare Advantage Plan.

This plan offers combined medical and prescription drug coverage as an alternative to the original Medicare program.

Part D is the Prescription Drug Plan.

It helps pay for your prescription medications.

Now let us look deeper into the various parts of Medicare.

Chapter 2

Making Sense of the Alphabet Soup of Medicare

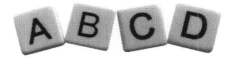

Part A: hospital insurance, Part B: medical insurance, Part C: Medicare Advantage Plan, Part D: Prescription Drug Plan.

How Does Original Medicare work?

Original Medicare is similar to a private fee-for-service plan. You receive a service and pay a fee. Medicare typically pays 80% of the total cost while you cover a 20% copay for Medicare-approved services after you have met your annual Part B deductible. Also, note that there is no limit to the 20% copay under original Medicare, so you should consider additional coverage through Part C, Medicare

Advantage Plan, and Part D, Prescription Drug Plan, or Medicare Supplement Plan.

Medicare Part A

Part A covers in-patient hospital care.

When hospitalized, you will have to normally pay a deductible for each 60 Day in-patient hospital stay.

Action Step

You can check Medicare.gov for the current deductible for each hospital stay during a 60-day period. There's also a copay for days 61–90, and a different copay for days 91–150. Days 91-150 is also commonly referred to as the lifetime reserve days.

Note: Coverage <u>ceases</u> after 150 days. You will be responsible for all costs.

In-patient psychiatric care, which usually has 190 days of a lifetime coverage, is also included. You can go to Medicare.gov or call 1-800-633-4227 for current copays and deductibles for your plan year.

Skilled Nursing Care: Days 1–20, no coinsurance. Days 21–100, coinsurance charged at a daily rate.

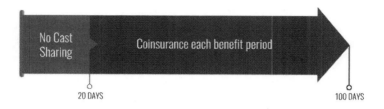

No Cast Sharing | Coinsurance each benefit period

20 DAYS   100 DAYS

Action Step:

For current copay for skilled nursing, days 21–100, call 1-800-633-4227 or go to Medicare.gov.

Home Healthcare is also covered. You typically will need to be certified to receive home healthcare benefits. Check with your primary care doctor. Hospice care for the terminally ill and individuals that have a life expectancy of 6 months or less is also covered.

Chapter 3

Medicare Part B

What is Medicare Part B coverage?
Medicare Part B covers certain doctor services, outpatient care, medical supplies, and preventative services.

Medicare Part B Benefits
Medical services and supplies covered by Medicare Part B include but not limited to:

- Doctor visits
- Laboratory tests
- X-rays
- Emergency and ambulance services
- Mental health services
- Durable medical equipment
- Preventive services such as flu shots and screenings
- Rehabilitation services

Note: Part B is optional. Some people that have other health coverage do not require Part B coverage, such as those who are 65+ years old and covered under an employer's health benefit plan. If they lose their employer health coverage due to retirement, they will be eligible for their Part B benefits without any penalty.

Action Step:

If you are currently covered under an employer health plan, check with your employer's human resources or benefits departments before you sign up for Part B to see if doing so will affect your employer's group health plan. Also ask if this is "creditable coverage."

Note: If you have employer group coverage you can delay getting Part B without penalty as long as your group health coverage is creditable coverage, meaning that the group coverage is as good as what Medicare benefits provide.

Medicare Part B Cost

Most people will receive Medicare Part A for free, but Part B is a premium service normally charged on a monthly basis. It come directly out of your social security check if you receive one, and otherwise you will be billed for the Part B premium.

Note: Part B premiums can change each year, and your Part B premium may be subject to an income-related adjustment. Medicare provides a chart that shows the current year's income limits so you can determine if you will have to pay a higher premium.

Action Step:

To see if you will have to pay an income-related adjustment for Part B, you can refer to the "Medicare and You" handbook or visit www.medicare.gov and search for income related adjustments. The adjustments may apply to single or married incomes.

Part B Deductible

Under the original Medicare's **Part B deductible**, you must pay all costs up to the Medicare-approved amount until you meet the yearly Part B deductible—only then will Medicare pay its share.

Note: Some Medicare Advantage Plans and Medigap Plans cover your yearly Part B deductible.

Part B Coinsurance

After you meet your deductible, you **pay 20%** of the Medicare-approved amount of the service if the doctor or health care provider accepts assignment. There's no yearly maximum for what you pay out-of-pocket under original Medicare.

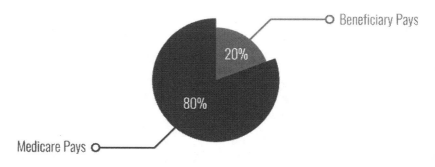

Action Step 1

Visit Medicare.gov or call 1-800-Medicare (1-800-633-4227). TTY users: 1-877-486-2048 for Medicare Part B deductible, and visit www.medicare.gov.

Action Step 2

You can also find out Part B premium costs at these same locations. If you're covered by an employer plan, check with your employer's benefits administrator about whether you should apply for Part B and if you will lose your employer group coverage if you do so. Weigh the costs and the benefits before you make any final decisions.

Action Step 3

Note: you do not need Part B to apply for Part D prescription drug coverage. You only need Part A to purchase Part D coverage. If you have employee group coverage, make sure you check with your human resources or benefits administrator before you add Part D coverage because it may affect your employee group coverage benefits.

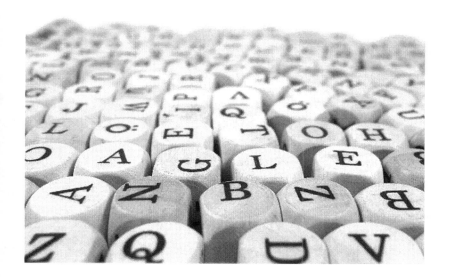

What is Assignment?

Knowing the meaning of "Assignment" is important when it comes to receiving Medicare benefits. If a doctor or other health care provider does not take a Medicare assignment, you may be responsible for the entire fee. So, "Assignment" is an agreement with your doctor, provider, or supplier——to accept the payment amount Medicare approves for the service and not to bill you for more than the Medicare deductible and coinsurance. If the Medicare Part B deductible applies, you must pay all costs until you meet the annual deductible before Medicare begins to pay its share. After your deductible is met, you typically pay 20% of the Medicare-approved amount for the service. You may also owe a copayment for certain outpatient services.

Who Is Eligible for Part B?

Anyone eligible for Medicare Part A is eligible for Medicare Part B— you must simply sign up for Part B and pay the Part B premium. If you are not eligible for Medicare Part A, you can qualify for Medicare Part B by meeting the following requirements: 65 years of age or older, a US citizen, or a permanent resident lawfully residing in the United States for 5 continuous years.

Note: You may also qualify for Medicare Part B enrollment through disability. If you are under 65 when receiving Social Security or Railroad Retirement Disability Benefits (RRDB), you will automatically be enrolled in Medicare Part A and Part B after 24 months of disability benefits. You may also qualify if you have end-stage renal disease (ESRD), ALS, or Lou Gehrig's disease.

Action Step

To see if a medical service is covered under Medicare Part B, ask your doctor or health care provider if it's medically necessary, which means any needed service or supply used to diagnose or treat medical conditions that meet accepted standards of medical practice. Your doctor or provider will be able to advise you if the service is covered by Medicare.

Part B Medical Insurance Covers:

- Doctors and other providers
- Ambulances
- Out-patient services
- X-rays
- Laboratory services
- Durable medical equipment
- Preventive services

Action Step

To see a complete listing of covered services under Part B, go to Chapter 5 or visit www.medicare.gov.

Medicare covers a broad range of services; however, it excludes certain types of care, treatment, and services.

Parts A and B Do Not Cover:

- Long-term care insurance, also known as custodial care
- Hearing aids
- Cosmetic surgery
- Dentures and most dental care
- Eye exams related to prescription eyeglasses

- Acupuncture
- Most care obtained outside the United States
- Most of the prescription drugs taken as an outpatient
- Most chiropractic services
- Routine foot care

Chapter 4

Eligibility and Enrollment

Medicare Part A

Let's look at how one becomes eligible for Medicare Part A and how to enroll.

One of the best parts of Medicare is that Part A is free for most people. To qualify, you simply need to meet a few requirements. The requirements are listed Below.

1. If you or your spouse have paid into Social Security for at least 10 years, Part A is free to you. Your Part A Medicare coverage will begin the first day of your birth month during the year that you turn 65. Three months before your 65th birthday, you should receive your Medicare card and enrollment packet that details your Part A benefits coverage and additional information on covered services.

2. If you are a citizen or a permanent resident of the United States.

3. If you currently receive or are eligible for Social Security or railroad retirement benefits.

4. You, your spouse, or ex-spouse receives Social Security benefits.

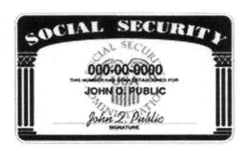

Here's an example of what a Medicare card looks like.

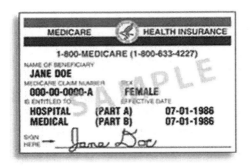

Now, what happens if you don't automatically receive an enrollment package for Part A?

If you are a US citizen or permanent resident of the United States and are age 65 or older, you can still enroll in Medicare Part A even if you have not reached your full Social Security retirement age. In other words, if you are older than 65 but you have not started withdrawing Social Security, you can still apply for Part A benefits.

If you receive railroad retiree benefits, you will be signed up automatically for Medicare Part A. If you are still working past age 65, you will still receive Part A employer coverage, but it will be your secondary insurance if you have coverage through an employer group plan.

Contact Medicare and request an enrollment packet at www.Medicare.gov or call 1-800-663-4227.

Part B

Let's look at your options. Part B coverage is optional. Anyone eligible for Medicare Part A qualifies for Medicare Part B by enrolling in and paying a monthly premium. If you are not eligible for Medicare Part A, you can qualify for Medicare Part B by meeting the following requirements: you must be 65 years or older, you must be a US citizen, or a permanent resident lawfully residing in the US for at least 5 continuous years.

Note: You may also qualify for Medicare Part B enrollment through disability. If you are under 65 when receiving Social Security or

Railroad Retirement (RRB) disability benefits, you will automatically be enrolled in Medicare Part A and Part B after 24 months of disability benefits. You may also qualify if you have end-stage renal disease (ESRD), ALS, or Lou Gehrig's disease.

Part B medical insurance helps to pay for your doctors and other providers, out-patient services, x-rays, laboratory services, durable medical equipment, ambulances, preventative services, supplies, and more. Keep in mind that you will pay a monthly premium for Part B coverage. The premium amount can change annually. You can check with Medicare online at Medicare.gov or call 1-800-633-4227 for current Part B premium rates.

You will have several opportunities to enroll for Part B coverage. Your first opportunity will be your initial enrollment period (IEP). There's a 7-month window to sign up, which begins 3 months before you turn age 65 and continues through the month of your 65th birthday and for 3 months following your 65th birthday month.

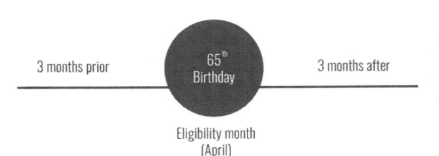

If you miss your initial enrollment period (**IEP**), you will be allowed to enroll during the **General Enrollment Period** from January 1 through March 30. However, a late enrollment penalty may apply. We will discuss this in more detail in later chapters.

What happens if you decide to work past age 65, and you continue to have employee health coverage? If you have health coverage through an employer group health plan, you have the option of delaying enrollment in Part B until you retire.

What if you retire after age 65 with employee group coverage?
Medicare will allow you an 8-month special enrollment period before applying for Part B coverage with a zero penalty. The enrollment begins on the date employer or union coverage ends.

If you are already receiving Social Security or railroad retiree benefits, Medicare will automatically sign you up for Part B coverage. You should receive your Medicare card within 60 days prior to your birth month, and your Part B coverage will begin the first day of the month of your 65th birthday. Also, note that Social Security will deduct your Part B premium from your Social Security check unless other arrangements are made.

Action Steps

What if I decide that I do not want to enroll in Medicare Part B?
Then you should follow the instructions provided in the Medicare enrollment package you received from Medicare.

If you do not receive your Part B enrollment package: Call the Social Security Administration at 1-800-633-4227 and request an enrollment package.

Keep this in mind especially if you do not apply for Medicare Part B when you first become eligible because you may face a late enrollment penalty of 10% for every year that you wait to enroll in Part B once your coverage ends, such as: if you fail to apply for Part B coverage when you turned age 65 during your **Initial Enrollment Period (IEP)** and you did not have employer group coverage.

Eligibility Due to Disability

If you are under age 65 and have been receiving Social Security benefits for a disability for 24 months, you will be automatically enrolled in Medicare. Example: Jane is 40 years old and was injured in car accident in which she sustained an injury that left her unable to work. She began receiving Social Security benefits, after the 24th month, she would be automatically enrolled in Medicare.

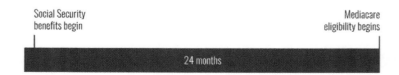

Social Security
benefits begin

Mediacare
eligibility begins

24 months

Chapter 5

What is Covered under the Part B Premium?

- You welcome to Medicare preventive visit
- Your annual wellness visit
- Tests (other than lab tests)
- Urgent care
- Shots, such as the – flu shot
- Hepatitis B and pneumococcal
- Surgical dressing services
- Telehealth
- Transplants and immunosuppressive drugs
- Speech language pathology services
- Second surgical pinions
- Prostate cancer screening
- Rural health clinics
- Sexually transmitted infections (STIs)
- Screenings and counseling
- Pulmonary rehabilitation
- Prosthetic and orthotic items
- Pneumococcal shot

- Smoking and tobacco-use cessation
- Counseling
- Prescription drugs (limited)
- Out-patient hospital services
- Out-patient medical and surgical services and supplies
- Occupational therapy
- Obesity screenings and counseling
- Physical therapy
- Mental health care (out-patient)
- Laboratory services
- Medical nutrition therapy services
- Cancer screenings
- Hepatitis C screening tests
- HIV screenings
- Home health services
- Kidney dialysis services and supplies
- Kidney disease education services
- Foot exams and treatment
- Hearing and balance exams
- Glaucoma tests
- Eyeglasses (limited)
- EKG or ECG (electrocardiogram screenings)
- Emergency departments
- Federal qualified health center (FQHC) services
- Diabetes self-management training
- Durable medical equipment (DME)

Note: Part B deductible applies to diabetes supplies. Visit Medicare.gov/supplier_directory to find a directory listing diabetes self-management training.

- Depression screening
- Defibrillator (implantable automatic)
- Continuous positive airway pressure (CPAP) therapy
- Concierge care
- Colonoscopy screenings
- Colorectal screenings
- Clinical research studies
- Chiropractor services (limited coverage)
- Cervical and vaginal screenings
- Chemotherapy
- Cardiovascular disease screenings
- Behavioral therapy
- Cardiac rehabilitation
- Breast cancer screenings
- Mammograms
- Bone mass measurements
- Bone density
- Blood work
- Ambulances
- Ambulatory surgical centers (out-patient surgery)
- Ambulatory services

Chapter 6

Types of Medicare Advantage Plans

Medicare Part C commonly known as (Medicare Advantage plans "MAPD" or "MA Plans").

Private insurance companies who are contracted with CMS, Centers for Medicare Services, provide these plans. An Advantage plan is another way to receive your benefits. There's a difference between Medicare Medigap plans and Advantage plans.

Under a MediGap plan, it pays a portion of your medical approved expenses after Medicare pays. Under a Medicare Advantage plan, the plan pays for your approved medical expenses subject to co-pays and deductibles. Medicare Advantage plans are often PPOs or HMOs and have a network of providers that may require a referral to see a specialist or other healthcare providers. Advantage plans often include extra benefits like dental, vision, chiropractic, acupuncture, discounts and reward programs. When you join an Advantage plan, you still have original Medicare, and your Medicare Advantage plan will be responsible for your Medicare approved Part A hospital and

Part B medical insurance benefits and they typically include Part D coverage at no additional cost.

HMO - Health Maintenance Organization

With an HMO plan, you will have a network of doctors, hospitals, and other medical providers. You select a PCP, a primary care physician from within the network. This doctor will be responsible for your care. If you need to have any tests or see a specialist, you would usually be required to get a referral from your primary care provider.

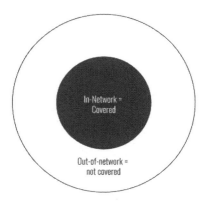

Action Step 1:

With a Medicare Advantage plan, you would normally have to use a network of providers to receive services. If you go outside of the network, you will usually have to pay 100% of the cost of the care.

An exception would be approval of the plan or emergency services while traveling.

Note: Medicare Advantage plans must cover all approved services that Medicare covers except hospice and some clinical research studies. Some plans cover this. You can check with plans in your local service area by visiting their individual websites, or refer to your Medicare & You Handbook.

Action Step 2

- Check to make sure that your primary care doctors and specialists are in the plan network.
- Check to see if your hospital choice is in the network.
- Check to see if your plan covers Part D, prescription drugs.
- Check plan ratings. Plans rated 3 and higher are recommended.

Also note: Medicare Advantage plans may offer some additional perks like **Free** gym membership, Dental, Vision, Chiropractic, Acupuncture, Hearing, and over-the-counter (OTC) benefits at no extra charge. Compare plan extras in your plan area.

PPO Plan

Preferred Provider Organization. Normally a PPO plan will have a network of doctors, hospitals, and other healthcare providers. This is known as the "preferred provider network." You can also go out of network for covered services and normally pay a higher cost. You have the flexibility to go to any doctor or hospital that accepts Medicare assignment with this type of Medicare Advantage plan.

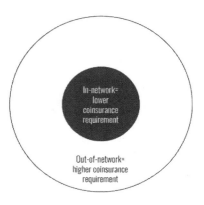

Action Step 1:

Check to see if your doctor, or specialist hospitals or other healthcare providers are in the preferred network so that you can save money. Check for premium cost; PPO plans normally charge a monthly premium, a yearly deductible, and co-pays for services within the PPO network and out of PPO network.

If the fees aren't too high, you may consider a Medicare Supplement plan or a Medicare Advantage plan. You can also go to Medicare.gov/pick –a-plan, or you can reference the Medicare & You Handbook for individual plans in your service area or visit the plan websites.

Special Needs Plan (SNP)

These plans are also known as **SNPS**. These plans are designed for individuals who have Medicare and Medicaid, or people with specific chronic or disabling conditions like chronic heart failure, ESRD (End-Stage Renal Disease), dementia, HIV/AIDS, and diabetes. The plan is very similar to an HMO plan. Normally you will have to stay within a network of doctors, hospitals, and other healthcare providers with the exception of emergency care.

You will normally pick a primary care doctor, a PCP, and may be required to have a referral to see a specialist or other healthcare provider. Prescription drugs Part D, are covered in these plans.

Action Step 1

Visit www.Medicare.gov/publications to view Your Guide to Medicare Special Needs Plans, SNPS, or got to Medicare.gov/find-a-plan. Most insurance companies will list their plan options on their websites. On the other hand, shop around because most SNP plans offer options that are not available in other Medicare Advantage plans.

Action Step 2:

You may qualify for a Special Needs Plan if you are in any low-income bracket and may receive extra help paying for prescription drugs, also known as **"low-income-subsidy" (LIS.)**

Action Step 3:

To see if you qualify for "**Extra Help with Prescription drugs**," go to: www.CMS.gov and look under "low-income-subsidy for Medicare prescription drug coverage" or call your local state Medicaid office to see if you qualify for extra help.

Note:

There are income limitations, proof of age or disability and accountable resources to be eligible for this program. To see these current limits, go to Medicare.gov or you can search under

- Specified low income Medicare beneficiary (SLMB) program
- Qualified Medicare Beneficiary (QMB) program
- Qualifying Individual (QI) program
- Qualified Disabled and Working Individual (QDWI) program

Action Step: Go online to www.ssi.gov for further information or to see if you qualify.

Private Fee for Services (PFFS)

This plan will allow you to see any doctor, hospital or health care provider that accepts Medicare, and the plan's payment terms and conditions. You normally do not need to pick a primary care doctor, and you do not need a referral to see a specialist. Part D, prescription drugs may be included, or you may have to purchase separate drug coverage.

Action Step:

Check with each individual plan in your plan service area and compare their terms of service and "Summary of Benefits." Verify that your Doctors and medical providers will accept the plans "Terms and conditions for payment" of provided services.

Refer to your Medicare & You Handbook for further information on plans in your service area.

Medicare and You Handbook

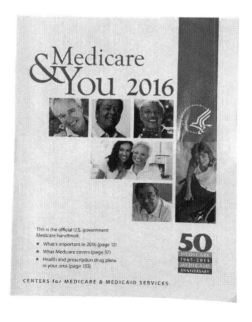

MSA, Medical Savings Account.

A combo plan that combines a high-deductible health plan with a bank account.

Visit www.Medicare.gov/publications for more information.

HMO Point of Service (HMOPOS)

These are HMO plans that may allow you to go out of network and pay a higher co-pay or a higher coinsurance cost.

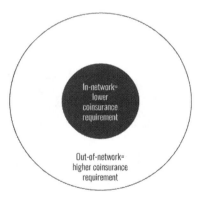

Chapter 7

How to Join a Medicare Advantage Plan, "Part C."

1. You will need to have **Part A** and **Part B**.

2. You must reside in a plan service area, which is normally the county of the plan that it services.

3. You are guaranteed acceptance with pre-existing conditions with one exception. If you have End-Stage Renal Disease (ESRD), then contact Medicare. They have special programs for this condition. You can also call 1-800-633-4227or go online at www.Medicare.gov/publications for more information.

4. You have to be a citizen or lawfully present in the United States. Note; most Medicare Advantage plans include Part D prescription drug coverage, so you may not need a separate drug plan. Check your individual plan. If you purchase a Part D drug plan after enrolling in a Medicare Advantage plan, you will be automatically disenrolled from your advantage plan, and you will have original Medicare and

partly coverage only, so be extra cautious when making changes after you join a Part C plan.

Note:

Advantage plans may include Part D prescription drug coverage at no additional cost. Some plans may charge monthly premiums, co-pays or coinsurance for only the services you use and not for the services that you don't use to help keep premiums lower. Some Medicare Advantage Plans offer zero premium plans and zero co-pays for some or a majority of services.

Also, if you would like to check out the quality of the plans and how Medicare rates particular plans, they publish ratings on Medicare.gov. Plans are rated from a 1-star to a 5-star, with a 5-star rated the highest.

Action Step

Check out plans in your service area by going to www.Medicare.gov for a listing of available plans. Check with local plans to see what extra services are provided such as gym memberships, dental, vision, etc. Note; some plans offer more choices and may provide different networks of doctors and medical providers. Some plans allow you to get services (out of network), but you may have to pay higher costs for these services. Make a list of the benefits that are important to you and shop around. A licensed insurance representative certified with Medicare can be a useful resource and save you time in your benefit search.

Chapter 8

Medicare Part D

Part D provides coverage for prescription drugs, and Medicare Part D is optional.

There are multitudes of coverage options, deductibles, co-pays, drugs covered, and insurance premium costs.

Private insurance companies sell all Part D plans. They are sold as a stand-alone drug plan or are included with a **Medicare Advantage Plan (MAPD.)**

When selecting a Part D prescription drug plan, every plan will include a **"Formulary."** The formulary is a listing of the drugs covered in the Part D drug plan. The listings will include the name of the drugs followed by a **"Tier"** number. The Tier structures are broken down into Tier 1, Tier 2, Tier 3, Tier 4, Tier 5, and sometimes Tier 6, depending on the plan you select, and can vary between plans. Point to remember: the higher the Tier, the higher the drug will cost you.

Here is an example of a typical formulary classification listing:

- A (**Tier 1**) drug would normally be classified as a **"Preferred Generic"** drug.

- A (**Tier 2**) would normally be classified as a **"Non-Preferred Generic"** drug.
- A (**Tier 3**) would normally be classified as a **"Name Brand"** drug.
- A (**Tier 4**) would normally be classified as a **"Non-Preferred Name Brand"** drug.
- A (**Tier 5**) would typically be higher priced like **"Injectable"** drugs.

Now that you have identified what drugs are included in your plan, their individual "Tier" classifications, how do you determine the drug costs?

Every Part D plan will have a **"Summary of Benefits."** The summary of benefits will list the co-pays or the cost for the tier classification of the drug that you are selecting. The summary of benefits will also list your Part D deductibles, if any. It will list any coverage limits, coverage gaps, and maximum out-of-pocket limits.

The benefit structure will help you to determine your drug costs for each particular drug that you are taking so that you can determine if the prescription drug plan meets your needs and budget.

Action Steps

- You can compare plan Formularies, premiums, and drug costs in your service by researching provider plans in your service area.

- You repeat these steps with each company you are comparing to determine the drug costs of the plan that fits your needs and your budget.

- When selecting a plan, make sure that your drugs are covered in the plan. You can do this by looking at the plan's prescription **Part D Formulary.** The Formulary will list all the drugs covered inside of the plan. After you verify that your drugs are covered in the plan, you can now determine the individual drug costs for the quantity and limits of those various drugs.

- Medicare has a website that you can compare your drug costs between individual plans in your service area. The website is www.medicare.gov/find-a-plan. You will enter the zip code for the service area you live in. The site will ask you a few questions and require you to list the drugs names, milligrams and quantity, and will provide a listing of all plan providers with costs in your plans service area.

Tier Reductions

Most Medicare drug plans list their drugs into different "tiers" on their prescription drug formularies. Drugs listed within these tiers will have different costs. A drug listed in a lower tier will normally cost you less than a drug in a higher tier. If your drug is listed in a higher tier and your doctor believes that you need that drug instead of a similar drug on a lower tier, you and your doctor can ask your plan for a tier exception to get a lower copayment. Note: Tier exception requests are not guaranteed.

Formulary Changes

Medicare drug plans can make changes to its formularies during the plan year. If the change includes a drug that you are currently taking, then your plan must do one of these:

- Provide written notice to you at least 60 days before the date the change becomes effective.

- At the time you request a refill, provide written notice of the change and provide you with a 60-day supply of the drug under the same plan rules as before the change.

Action Step

Tier Exception: Ask your physician, to write a letter to the service plan and explain why you need a tier reduction. If the plan approves your request, you could be paying a lower co-pay and save money on your drug cost.

Also note: *Formulary change*, Medicare drug plans can change their formulary during the plan year. If this change affects the drug you are taking, the plan will notify you of the change 60 days before the change. You will be allowed a 60-day to a 90-day supply when you get your refill. This will give your doctor time to step you into a new drug during this transition. It is critical that you remember when you are Medicare eligible, Medicare requires you to have drug coverage, commonly known as Part D. If you do not get drug coverage when eligible, you may have to pay a late enrollment penalty fee. The late enrollment penalty is calculated at 1% of the nationally based premium, multiplied by the number of months you are eligible.

Here's an Example of How a Part D Penalty is applied.

Jane was in good health when she became eligible for Part D. Because she was not taking any prescription drugs at the time, she chose not to enroll. A year later, Jane's health status changed, and she was diagnosed with high blood pressure and high cholesterol and had to start taking prescription drugs daily to manage her condition. During the next enrollment period, Jane enrolled in a stand-alone prescription drug plan.

At this point, Jane has gone without credible coverage for 12 months' period. Her penalty would be calculated by 1% of the nationally based premium multiplied by the number of months that she was eligible. Her new premium surcharge is permanent, and that is why it is important to consider the penalty carefully if you are planning to delay Part D enrollment. If you purchase a Medicare supplement plan, you should consider looking at purchasing a Part D prescription drug plan, or, if you purchase Medicare Part C Advantage Plan, it may already include Part D coverage at no additional cost.

Action Steps:

How to Avoid a Part D Penalty.

- Purchase Part D coverage when you first become eligible.

- Purchase a Part C Medicare Advantage plan. It will normally include Part D coverage.

- If you purchase a Medicare "Medigap" plan, consider purchasing a Medicare Part D prescription drug plan at the same time to avoid penalties in the future.

- You can also prevent the penalty by showing proof of credible coverage from an employer or union health plan if you had coverage before turning age 65 or after obtaining the age of 65. You could also have this coverage under a spouse's employer plan, if you had coverage through your spouse's employer group coverage. This would also qualify as credible drug coverage. You can check with your employer's plan administrator to verify that you had credible coverage.

Medicare Part D Insurance Coverage Options:

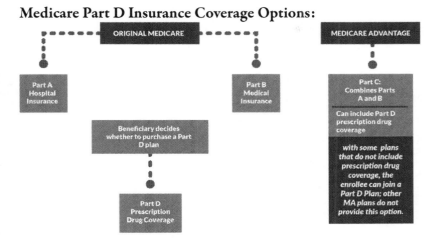

Part D Action Steps:

Step 1

Initial Enrollment Period Is when you turn 65, you can enroll in a Part D plan during the 7 month period that starts 3 months before you turn 65 and continues through the 3 months after you turned 65 years of ages.

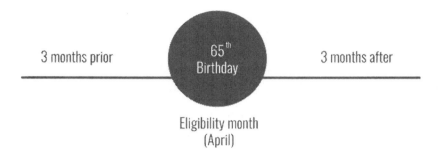

3 months prior   65th Birthday   3 months after

Eligibility month
(April)

Step 2

If you joined a **Medicare Advantage Plan (MAPD)**, it would normally include Part D coverage. You can check Medicare Part C plans in your service area to ensure that they do include Medicare Part D coverage. You can go to medicare.gov or you can visit individual insurance company websites or contact a local Medicare specialist in your area who can do this work for you.

Also note: you may owe a late Part D enrollment penalty at any time after your initial enrollment period is over. If there is a period of 63 or more days in a row when you don't have Part D credible prescription drug coverage, you may be subject to a penalty.

What to Do If You Receive a Penalty Notice.

You can contact your plan about the drug coverage if you believe that you should not be charged a penalty and ask the plan to assist you in sending a letter to help you avoid the penalty.

Obtain proof of **creditable coverage** from your previous employer to show proof of coverage to avoid a penalty.

"**Creditable prescription drug coverage**-Prescription drug coverage (for example, from an employer or union) that's expected to pay, on average at least as much as Medicare's standard prescription drug coverage."

Chapter 9

Medicare Part D and the "Coverage Gap" also known as the Infamous (Donut Hole.)

In 2016, minimum a plan can offer:

1. The Part D plan member pays the first $360 as an annual Part D deductible.

2. **"Initial Coverage Limit"** begins. The member pays 25 percent, and the Part D plan pays 75 percent of the drugs' costs up to a combined amount of $3,310 in drug costs, including the annual deductible.

3. After reaching $3,310 in total drug costs, you enter the **"Coverage Gap,"** what is known as the (Donut Hole). The member pays 45% of the plan costs for covered brand-name drugs and 58% for covered generic drugs in the Coverage Gap.

4. After you and the plan have exceeded $4,850 in total out-of-pocket costs, you enter what is known as **"Catastrophic Coverage."**

At this point, you will be responsible for paying the greater of 5% or $2 and 95 cents for generic drugs and $7 and 40 cents for all other drugs through the end of the plan year.

Note: Under the 2010 health care reform law, Medicare will eventually close the Medicare Part D donut hole. You can visit www.medicare.gov to check out the current Part D deductible, initial coverage limits, coverage gap, and catastrophic coverage amounts; these amounts change annually.

Part D Minimum Requirements

2016

Deductible	$360
Initial Coverage	$3,310
Out-of-Pocket (OOP) threshold	$4,850

Main copay (Catastrophic portion of benefit)

- Generic/Preferred Drug $2.95
- All other drugs $7.40
  Under the Affordable Care Act (ACA)

The standard Part D benefit now includes coverage in the Coverage Gap, (donut hole) under the Affordable Care Act (ACA). Before 2011, the standard benefit did not include coverage between the initial coverage limit and the level of spending at which the OOP threshold was met, i.e., where the catastrophic coverage commenced. In 2016, there will be a 42% plan benefit (58% retiree-paid coinsurance) for generic drugs and a 5% plan benefit for brand drugs.

There continues to be a separately calculated 50% brand drug discount provided by the manufacturer of the brand drug. The combination of the 5% plan benefit and 50% brand discount results in 45% retiree-paid coinsurance for brand drugs is 2016. The total amount of spending required to reach the OOP threshold and catastrophic coverage will depend on whether spending is on generic drugs, brand drugs, or a combination. By 2020, the Part D coverage gap will be completely phased out through the combination of the additional Part D benefit and brand discount.

Chapter 10

What is Medicare Supplement "Medigap?"

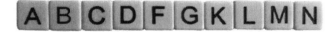

Medicare Supplement also known as "**Medigap Plans**" is a private health insurance contract designed to supplement original Medicare by covering some or all the gaps in original Medicare.

This means that it helps to pay for some of the improved Medicare costs that would normally be your responsibility, such as coinsurance, copayments, and deductibles.

The major differences between Medigap insurance plans may be the premium cost charged for the same plan, and any additional benefits they may include outside of what Medicare covers.

Advantages of "Medigap" Plans

Medigap plans provide more freedom and flexibility when choosing your care options. With the exception of Medicare Select policies, you can use any medical provider or services that accept original Medicare. In other words, your Medigap plan does not require you to use a network of providers.

No referral is required to see a specialist.

Provides continuous coverage as long as you pay your premiums. "Guaranteed renewable."

Some of the gap plans cover additional benefits. An example would be a plan that offers additional coverage while traveling outside the United States, gym memberships, discount plans, and other services.

Disadvantages of "Medigap" Plans

More expensive compared to Medicare Advantage plans.

Premiums subject to increase annually.

Medigap plans do not include prescription drug coverage. You will need to purchase a stand-alone PDP drug plan.

If you purchase a Medigap plan outside of your "open enrollment period," you will have to qualify through Medical underwriting.

Some insurance companies may offer a **High-Deductible Plan F** in some states. By choosing this option, you would be responsible for paying all Medicare-covered costs, copayments, coinsurance, and deductibles up to the annual deductible amount before your policy pays. This option bodes well for individuals that are in good health. The premiums are much lower in the High-Deductible Plan F option, and the premium savings could be substantial over time.

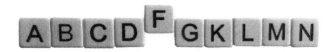

Now, let's look at the <u>Gaps</u> in Part A and Part B.

Part A Hospital Insurance Gaps

You will have a per benefit period deductible before Medicare pays your part A benefit. This applies annually during each benefit period.

There will also be a daily hospital coinsurance payments after you have met your deductible. During the first 60 days, Medicare will pay 100 percent of hospitalization costs. However, you will have to pay a daily copayment between days 61 through day 90, and, if your hospital stays go beyond 90 days, you will pay a higher co-pay days 91 through 150 days of the hospitalization.

Lifetime Reserve. Once you have used your lifetime reserve of 150 days of hospitalization, Medicare pays no benefits, and you would be responsible for all costs.

There are daily coinsurance payments for **Skilled Nursing Care (SNC).** When you qualify for skilled nursing, Medicare will cover 100% of the first 20 days of care. However, you will pay a daily co-pay from days 21 through day 100. After day 100, Medicare pays no benefit.

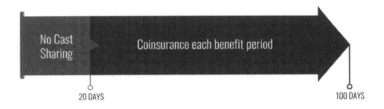

Home Healthcare is not covered for care that is provided on more than a part-time or intermittent basis. It does not cover if the home healthcare does not include skilled nursing care or [occupational or physical] care.

Part B Medical Expense Insurance Gaps

-    You will be responsible for paying an **Annual Deductible** for Medicare Part B medical covered services.

- **Coinsurance** - You will be responsible for a **20 percent** coinsurance for approved charges. Medicare will pay the remaining 80 percent of covered charges.

- When there is any charges above the Medicare approved amount for physicians and other services provided, Medicare will pay 80% and you will be responsible for up to the **15%** of the <u>limiting charge</u>.

Note:

Under Medicare, there is no-limit to the out-of-pocket costs that you can incur. For example, a hospital stay that lasts 150 days or longer would cost over forty-nine thousand dollars out of pocket, this is why I would recommend looking into a Medicare supplement, (Medigap) insurance plan, or a Medicare Advantage plan (MAPD) to protect you from these potential high out-of-pocket costs. Also, these costs are expected to Increase annually.

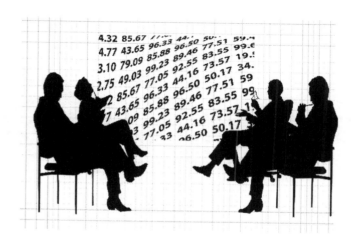

Now that we know some of the Gaps that MediGap plans may cover, let's look at what Medicare Supplement "Medigap" Plans <u>Do Not</u> Cover.

Medicare Supplement (MediGap) Plans
<u>Will Not</u> cover the following medical services

- Prescription drugs.
- Dental.
- Vision.
- Eyeglasses, with the exception of cataract surgery.
- Hearing aids.
- Medicare Advantage plans.
- Medicaid.
- Employer or union plans.
- Federal employees' health benefit plans and programs.
- Veterans' benefits.
- Tri-care.
- Long-term care - custodial care.
- Indian health services.
- Tribal and Indian health plans.
- Qualified plans.
- Private duty nursing.

When Can You Buy a Medigap Policy?

There are three times you can purchase a policy.

1. Medicare Supplement (Medigap) open enrollment is when you first become eligible. It begins when you are 65 or older and enrolled in Medicare Part B. Enrollment lasts for 6 months, starting on the first day of the month you enroll in your Part B.

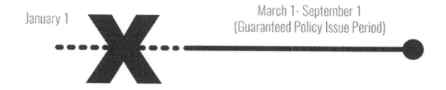

January 1

March 1- September 1
(Guaranteed Policy Issue Period)

Note: This period may begin when you <u>turn age 65</u> and age into Medicare and enroll in Part B or when you <u>Retire</u> or <u>lose your Union or Group coverage</u> at an age older than 65 from an employer/Union group health plan and enroll in Part B.

The main reason open enrollment is the best time to buy a Medicare Supplement (Medigap) policy is because insurance companies can't use medical underwriting to qualify you. You have **Guaranteed Issue Rights**. They cannot refuse to sell you any policy it currently sells.

They can't make you wait for coverage to start with one exception: If you have been without coverage or had a lapse of 63+ days, you may be subject to a 6-month waiting period. The insurance company can look back 6 months into your medical history and may require a 6-month waiting period on pre-existing medical conditions.

If you have a 6-month waiting period for a pre-existing health condition, you will still have original Medicare coverage during this waiting period.

2. If you currently have a Medicare Advantage plan and your plan is not renewing or leaving the plan service area, Medicare will provide you with a guaranteed issue right to purchase a Medigap plan in the county in which you reside.

3. If you have employer or union group coverage including Cobra that is ending, you have a guaranteed issue rights. Coverage will not start until you sign up for your Part B.

Other conditions provide guaranteed issue rights. You can check with www.medicare.gov for all other conditions that may apply for a complete list.

Also note; under **Guaranteed Issue Rights**, Medigap insurance companies must provide the following:

- Must sell you a policy; policies may be limited.
- Cover pre-existing conditions, regardless of health conditions.

- Can't charge you more based on your health or your pre-existing conditions.
- You <u>cannot</u> own a Medicare supplement plan and a Medicare Advantage plan at the same time.
- You can, however, purchase a separate stand-alone Part D prescription drug plan to go with a Medicare Supplement Medigap plan.

How Do You Compare Medicare Supplement "Medigap" Plans?

Since plans are standardized, it's much easier to compare one company plan to another.

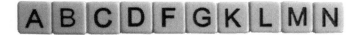

Premiums can vary between companies for the same plans, so it pays to compare prices and select the plan that suits your budget and provides the coverage options you are looking for.

Medigap Plan F

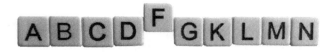

Plan F is one of the more popular plans, and it is the most comprehensive plan available.

Plan F covers 100% of:

- Medicare Part A coinsurance and hospital costs (up to an additional 365 days after Medicare benefits are used.
- Medicare Part B coinsurance or copayment
- Blood (first 3 pints)
- Part A hospice care coinsurance or copayment
- Part A deductible
- Part B deductible
- Part B excess charges
- Foreign travel emergency **80%** (up to plan limits)

High Deductible Plan F

Some plans offer a **High-Deductible Plan F** option. This plan offers a lower monthly premium cost. Under this option, you will pay for all Medicare-covered costs until you reach your annual deductible amount before your Plan pays. After you reach your annual deductible, the plan pays the same as a **Plan F** pays. This may be a good option for someone who is in good health and wants a lower premium cost.

Note: The deductible may change on an annual basis. However, the premiums are historically lower than the Plan F premiums.

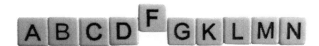

Plan N

Plan N is another attractive option for individuals who do not mind paying a little out-of-pocket. Plan N pays 100% of your Part B coinsurance , except for copayments up to $20 for some office visits and up to $50 for an emergency room visit that does not result in an inpatient hospital admission.

A B C D F G K L M N

The following chart is a breakdown of coverage options with Medicare Supplement "Medigap" plans:

Medicare Supplement Insurance (Medigap) plans

Benefits	A	B	C	D	F*	G	K	L	M	N
Medicare Part A coinsurance and hospital costs (up to an additional 365 days after Medicare benefits are used)	100%	100%	100%	100%	100%	100%	100%	100%	100%	100%
Medicare Part B coinsurance or copayment	100%	100%	100%	100%	100%	100%	50%	75%	100%	100%
Blood (first 3 pints)	100%	100%	100%	100%	100%	100%	50%	75%	100%	100%
Part A hospice care coinsurance or copayment	100%	100%	100%	100%	100%	100%	50%	75%	100%	100%
Skilled nursing facility care coinsurance			100%	100%	100%	100%	50%	75%	100%	100%
Part A deductible		100%	100%	100%	100%	100%	50%	75%	100%	100%
Part B deductible			100%		100%					
Part B excess charges					100%	100%				
Foreign travel emergency (up to plan limits)			80%	80%	80%	80%			80%	80%
							Out-of-pocket limit in 2015			
							$4,940	$2,470		

Action Steps:

- The best time to enroll in a Medigap plan is during your open enrollment period. This is the 6-month period beginning from the first day of the month that you are 65 years old or older and enrolled in the Medicare Part B plan.

- You will have **Guaranteed Issue Rights**. This means that the insurance is prohibited from using medical underwriting regardless of your healthcare or your past medical history. If you do not purchase the first time you are eligible, you will have to go through medical underwriting.

- **Note:** Some states may allow the insurance company to delay benefits on any pre-existing conditions for up to 6 months. Check with your agent or the insurance company you are applying for if the company has pre-existing conditions. If this becomes an issue for you, then look into Medicare Advantage plans because they accept all pre-existing conditions with the exception of "End-Stage Renal Disease" (ESRD.)

- **Guaranteed Renewability**. All Medigap plans are issued with a guaranteed renewable clause. The insurance company cannot cancel your policy regardless of health status. They can only cancel your policy for non-payment of premiums.

- If you currently have an employer or a union group coverage, you should consider delaying enrolling in Part B coverage. Your "open enrollment" will not begin until you enroll in Part B. When you enroll in Part B, you will have a 6-month period to purchase a Medigap or a Medicare Advantage plan, and the plan coverage will start on the first day of the month you become eligible. You could also check with your employer benefits department and they can advise you on your options while employed and what your options are and how they affect your current group coverage. This is very important because you don't want to upset the employer group coverage benefits by enrolling in Part B too early.

- You need to have Part A and Part B to buy a Medicare supplement "Medigap" policy.

- Each policy covers one person.

- You are going to pay a separate premium to a private insurance company and continue to pay your Part B premiums for Medicare.

- When comparing plans, all plans are standardized. That means a plan with insurance company A will be the same with insurance company B. The only difference will be the premiums, pre-existing conditions, waiting periods, and extra benefits like free gym memberships included with your plan.

- Compare plans. Contact a local licensed Medicare Agent to help you select the best plan based on your needs. It won't cost you anything extra to work with a licensed agent. I would recommend that you work with an agent who is licensed for both Medicare Advantage Plans and Medicare Supplement (Medigap) plans. This way you will get an unbiased comparison of both plans.

- Go to www.medicare.gov/find-a-plan. They have a listing of insurance companies and plans in your service area. You could also request a free booklet called "Choosing a Medigap Policy." The number to call is 1-800-633-4227, and request to have a book mailed to you.

- You can contact your local State Insurance Department for a listing of Insurance Companies licensed to sell Medigap plan.

- You can also contact your local State Insurance Health Program (SHIP) for a listing of Medigap plans in your service area.

- When you purchase a Medigap plan, you will need to buy a separate **stand-alone Part D** prescription drug plan. Go to www.medicare.gov/find-a-plan or call a local Medicare-certified licensed insurance professional to help you select the plan that best fits your needs and budget.

"The best advice I ever got was that knowledge is power and to keep reading."

David Bailey

Chapter 11

Enrollment Dates

Initial enrollment period (I-E-P): 3 months before you turn 65, the month you turn 65, 3 months after you turn 65. Also, if you retire after age 65 and your employer-sponsored coverage ends, you will have 2 months to enroll after your employer plan ends.

Under Medicare supplement, you can apply at any time during the year. You may apply outside the Medicare open enrollment period. Medicare supplement open enrollment starts on the first day of the month in which you turn 65 or with your Part B effective date. You must be enrolled in both Part A and Part B. The Medicare supplement open enrollment period lasts for 6 months. You are guaranteed a policy and are not subject to underwriting.

Note: Under a Medicare supplement policy, after your open enrollment period has ended, you will have to undergo underwriting to qualify for a policy. Every year after you first become eligible, you are eligible for general enrollment periods.

Enrollment Periods

Pre-Enrollment Period:
October 1 - October 14

Annual Election Period (A.E.P):
October 15 - December 7

Annual Dis-Enrollment Period (A.D.P):
January 1 - February 14

Special Election Period (S.E.P):
February 15 - October 14, if you qualify.

Here are more details about the Annual Election Period (A.E.P.). Between October 1 and October 14, you can look at various plans in your service area. However, you cannot sign up for a plan until October 15. Between October 15 and December 7, you can enroll in a plan. When you enroll in a new Medicare Part C or Part D plan, this action will automatically disenroll you from an existing Medicare plan, if you currently have a plan. An exception would be; if you're in a Medicare supplement plan, you will have to call and cancel that plan on January 1 of that following year. When you select a plan during the annual enrollment, your plan will not be effective until January 1 of the following year, so you will maintain the same benefits in the current plan that you have through December 31 of that plan year.

Also note: during the Annual Enrollment, you can join a Medicare Advantage plan, only if you have Part A and your Part B. You normally have to be a resident of the county you are applying for, and you normally have to reside in the county for at least 6 months and 1 day in the plan service area each calendar year. Individuals that travel, or, who live part-time in one state and live part-time in another state commonly referred to as "snowbirds." You will qualify as long as you live 6 months and 1 day in that plan area, you will be eligible for a Medicare Advantage plan. Some plans offer an <u>exception</u> if you are going to be out of the plan service area of the country for an extended period of time. Check with the plan that you are applying for to see if they offer this option. The only medical questions that can be asked when signing up for a Medicare Advantage plan is: **Do you have End Stage Renal Disease (ESRD)?** This would be the only medical question that could disqualify you from the (**MAPD**) plan. Medicare has a plan for those individuals. Contact Medicare directly for your options. Also, if you have a Medicare supplement plan, by joining a Medicare Advantage plan will automatically disenroll you from your Part D prescription drug plan, if you currently have a Part D drug plan.

Action Steps

- October 1st thru October 14th you can compare plans in your service area, but you can't make any changes.

- October 15th thru December 7th you can switch from one Medicare Advantage Plan or drug plan and enroll in another plan. The changes will become effective on January 1st of the new calendar year.

- If you are happy with your current plan, then you will not have to make any changes, you will be automatically re-enrolled in your current plan.

- If you are changing a Medigap plan, you may be subject to the plans underwriting. Check with the plan you are applying.

Annual Dis-Enrollment Period [A-D-P]: Between January 1 and February 14, you could disenroll from the Medicare Advantage plan or you could disenroll from a Medicare plan. You can also purchase your Medicare supplement plan and purchase a separate drug plan during the annual disenrollment period, or you can go back to the original Medicare and purchase a different drug coverage under the Part D prescription drug plan.

Here is more information regarding the special enrollment period between February 15th and October 14th. It is a qualifying event, more commonly known as an S-E-P. Typically, if you moved out of the plan's service area, you will have a special election period. You can enroll in a new plan. If you lose other credible prescription drug coverage, if you live in an institution like a nursing home, if you have Medicaid or Medi-Cal, you have an open enrollment period. Or, if you qualify for extra help with drugs, typically known as LIS, extra help with prescription drugs, you may legible for special enrollment periods throughout the year as well.

Chapter 12

What is Medicare Assignment under Original Medicare?

This would depend on whether your healthcare provider, doctor, or supplier accepts **assignment**. What is assignment? This means your healthcare provider, doctor, or supplier agrees or is required by law to accept Medicare approved amount as full payment for covered services. What if a provider, doctor, or supplier doesn't accept assignment? Non-participating providers who have not signed an agreement to accept assignment for all Medicare covered services can still accept assignment for services they provide.

Note: You may have to pay the entire bill at the time you receive the services, you may have to submit your own claim to Medicare, and you will need to use **Medicare form #CMS-1490S** to get reimbursed, or you can go to medicare.gov/medicare-online-forms to get the document. You may also be charged more than the normal Medicare approved amount and pay a high coinsurance. There is a limit called the limiting charge (but it does not apply to some supplies of durable medical equipment). Make sure that you check with your health provider or insurance provider for Medicare.

Note: under private contracts, if you choose a doctor or healthcare provider that does not provide services for Medicare and you sign a written private contract, Medicare will not pay for the services you received under this private contract even if it's a Medicare-covered service. Therefore, check with your Medicare provider to ensure that this will be covered, or it would be something you would be paying for out-of-pocket.

Chapter 13

Plan Ratings

Plans can be rated from 1-star to a 5-star. A 5-star plan is the highest rating possible. A plan with a 3-star rating is considered average, and it is recommended that you do not select a plan with a lower rating than 3 stars. 5-star plans have enrollment periods that extend beyond the normal annual enrollment dates. You can enroll between the dates of December 8 through November 30 each year. Also, note that you can only use 1 special enrollment period during this time frame if you do enroll in a 5-star plan during December 8 through December 30. To locate a 5-star plan in your service area or to locate individual star ratings, go to medicare.gov/find-a-plan.

FREE BONUS:
JOIN ME FOR FREE VIDEO TRAINING

Register right now to join me for Free Bonus Video Training. I will be covering Medicare Basics, Medicare Part C, Medicare Part D and Medicare Supplement (Medigap) plans.
Visit htttp://www.howtonavigatemedicare.com

Chapter 14

Medicare Costs for 2016

Part A Costs

For most people, Part A is free. You normally will not pay a monthly premium for Medicare Part A (Hospital Insurance) coverage if you or your spouse paid Medicare taxes while working for a period of (10 years) or (40 quarters.) This is what is called "premium-free Part A." Some people will automatically get Medicare Part A (Hospital Insurance). If you have to purchase Part A, you'll pay up to $411 each month.

You can get premium-free Part A at 65 if the following applies:

- You already get retirement benefits from Social Security or the Railroad Retirement Board.
- You're eligible to get Social Security or Railroad benefits but haven't filed for them yet.
- You or your spouse had Medicare-covered government employment.
- If you're under 65, you can get premium-free Part A if:

- You have Social Security disability benefits for 24 months
- You got Railroad Retirement Board disability benefits for 24 months.
- You have End-Stage-Renal-Disease (ESRD) and meet certain requirements.

In the majority of cases, if you purchase Part A, you must also have Medicare Part B (Medical Insurance) and pay monthly premiums for both.

Action Step:

Contact Social Security for more information about the Part A premium. www.socialsecurity.gov

Part B Costs

Some people will automatically receive Medicare Part B (Medical Insurance), and some people need to sign up for
Part B.

Action Step:

- To sign up for Part B you can sign up online at Social Security- www.socialsecurity.gov/medicareonly
- Visit your local Social Security office.

- Call Social Security at 1-800-772-1213. TTY users should call 1-800-325-0778.
- If you worked for a railroad, call the RRB at 1-877-772-5772.
- Complete an Application for Enrollment in Part B (CMS-40B).
- You can also obtain this form and instructions in Spanish. Remember, you must already have Part A to apply for Part B.
- Apply online at Social Security. www.socialsecurity.gov/medicare

If you don't sign up for Part B when you're first eligible, you may have to pay a late enrollment penalty.

How much does Part B cost?

Part B premiums

You pay a premium each month for Part B. If you get Social Security, Railroad Retirement Board, or Office of Personnel Management benefits, your Part B premium will be automatically deducted from your benefit payment. If you don't get these benefit payments, you'll get a bill.

Most people will pay the standard premium amount. However, if your modified adjusted gross income as reported on your IRS tax return from 2 years ago is above a certain amount, you may pay an

Income Related Monthly Adjustment Amount (IRMAA). IRMAA is an extra charge added to your premium.

The standard Part B premium amount is $121.80 (or higher depending on your income). However, most people who get Social Security benefits will continue to pay the same Part B premium amount as they paid in 2015. This is because there wasn't a cost-of-living increase for 2016 Social Security benefits. You'll pay a different premium amount if:

- You enroll in Part B for the first time in 2016.
- You don't get Social Security benefits.
- You're directly billed for your Part B premiums.
- You have Medicare and Medicaid, and Medicaid pays your premiums. (Your state will pay the standard premium amount of $121.80.)
- Your modified adjusted gross income as reported on your IRS tax return from 2 years ago is above a certain amount.

If you're in 1 of these 5 groups on the next page, here's what you'll pay:

If your yearly income in 2014 (for what you pay in 2016) was			
File individual tax return	File joint tax return	File married & separate tax return	You pay (in 2016)
$85,000 or less	$170,000 or less	$85,000 or less	$121.80
above $85,000 up to $107,000	above $170,000 up to $214,000	Not applicable	$170.50
above $107,000 up to $160,000	above $214,000 up to $320,000	Not applicable	$243.60
above $160,000 up to $214,000	above $320,000 up to $428,000	above $85,000 and up to $129,000	$316.70

above $214,000	above $428,000	above $129,000	$389.80

Part B Deductible & Coinsurance Costs

You pay $166 per year for your Part B deductible. After your deductible is met, you typically pay 20% of the Medicare-approved amount for most doctor services (including most doctor services while you're a hospital inpatient), outpatient therapy, and durable medical equipment.

Note:
In 2016, there may be limits on physical therapy, Occupational therapy and speech language pathology services. If so, there may be exceptions to these limits.

Medicare 2016 costs at a glance

If you choose not to purchase a Medicare Advantage (Part C) or Medicare Supplement (Medigap) insurance plan, it will be important to know what your Medicare Part A and/or Part B benefit costs for people with Medicare only. The following chart displays your 2016 costs.

2016 costs at a glance	
Part A premium	Most people don't pay a monthly premium for Part A (sometimes called "premium-free Part A"). If you buy Part A, you'll pay up to $411 each month. Calculate my premium.
Part A hospital inpatient deductible and coinsurance	You pay: • $1,288 deductible for each benefit period • Days 1-60: $0 coinsurance for each benefit period • Days 61-90: $322 coinsurance per day of each benefit period • Days 91 and beyond: $644 coinsurance per each "lifetime reserve day" after day 90 for each benefit period (up to 60 days over your lifetime) • Beyond lifetime reserve days: all costs.

Part B premium	Most people pay $104.90 each month.
Part B deductible and coinsurance	$166 per year. After your deductible is met, you typically pay 20% of the Medicare-approved amount for most doctor services (including most doctor services while you're a hospital inpatient), outpatient therapy, and durable medical equipment.
Part C premium	The Part C monthly premium varies by plan. Compare costs for specific Part C plans.
Part D premium	The Part D monthly premium varies by plan (higher-income consumers may pay more). Compare costs for specific Part D plans.

Note: For a hospital stay up to 150 days, it could cost somewhere in the neighborhood of $49,000 and if you were to exceed your lifetime reserve days, you would be responsible for all costs.

Costs for Medicare drug coverage

Your actual drug plan costs will vary depending on:

- The prescription drugs you use
- The drug plan you select
- Whether get your drugs at a pharmacy in your plan's network or out-of-network,

You may have to make these payments throughout the year in a Medicare prescription drug plan:

- Premium
- Annual deductible
- Copayments or coinsurance
- Costs in the coverage gap (Donut Hole)
- Costs if you get Extra Help
- Costs if you have to pay a late enrollment penalty.
- Whether the drugs you use are covered in your plan's formulary.

Action Steps:

- Research the plans you're interested in to get more details. If you have limited income and resources, your state may help you to pay for Part A and/or Part B. You may also qualify for

Extra Help to pay for your Medicare prescription drug coverage.

- Medicare Savings Programs (MSP) - programs in your state that help pay for your Medicare premiums, your Medicare Part A (hospital insurance) and Medicare Part B (medical insurance) deductibles, coinsurance, and copayments, and Medicare prescription drug coverage costs.

Medicaid, a joint federal and state program that helps with medical costs like nursing home care and personal care services, for some people with limited income and resources, you may qualify for extra help from Medicare to pay the costs of Medicare prescription drug coverage if you meet certain income and resource limits. Contact your local Medicaid office in your state.

Glossary

Medicare acronym reference guide

A.E.P- annual election period

Assignment - Health care provider agrees to accept Medicare's approved amount as full payment for Services.

Benefit Period - Under Medicare Part A, the benefit period begins on the day you are admitted to a hospital or skilled nursing facility and ends 60 days after you are discharged. If she or he is not readmitted to a hospital or skilled nursing facility within that time.

CMS - Centers for Medicare and Medicaid.

Coinsurance - Cost-sharing whereby the recipient pays a percentage of the cost of services, and the benefit program or insurance pays the rest.

Copayment - The recipient of the health care pays a flat fee for each covered service, and the benefit plan pays the remainder of charges.

Creditable prescription drug coverage -Prescription drug coverage (for example, from an employer or union) that's expected to pay, on average at least as much as Medicare's standard prescription drug coverage.

ESRD - End-stage renal disease.

Formulary - The list of drugs covered by an outpatient prescription drug plan.

G.E.P - General enrollment period.

Guaranteed renewable - A policy cannot be terminated or non-renewed except for non-payment of premium or material misrepresentation.

HMO - Health maintenance organization.

I.C.E.P - Initial coverage election (enrollment) period.

I.E.P - Initial election (enrollment) period, a seven-month period starting with the first day of the third month prior to the month an individual turns age 65, and extending to the last day of the month after the individual turns age 65.

I.E.P - Part D: initial enrollment period for Part D.

Life time reserve days - In Original Medicare, these are additional days that Medicare will pay for when you're in a hospital for more than 90 days. You have a total of 60 reserve days that can be used during your lifetime. For each lifetime reserve day, Medicare pays all covered costs except for a daily coinsurance.

LIS - Low-income subsidies "extra help" a program to help people with limited income and resources pay Medicare prescription drug program costs.

M.A.D.P - Medicare Advantage dis-enrollment period.

MA-only - Medicare Advantage plan without prescription drug.

M.A.P.D - MAPD: Medicare Advantage plan with prescription drugs.

Medicaid - Joint federal and state program that helps with medical costs for some people with limited income and resources. Medicaid programs vary from state to state, but most health care costs are covered if you qualify for both Medicare and Medicaid.

Medical - Also known as Medicaid in California.

Medicare Advantage Plan (Part C) - A type of health care plan offered by private insurance companies that contract with Medicare to provide you with all your Medicare Part A and Part B benefits. Medicare Advantage plans include Health Maintenance

Organizations, Preferred Provider Organizations, Private Fee-for-Service Plans, Special Needs Plans, and Medicare Savings Account Plans. If you're enrolled in a Medicare Advantage Plan, Medicare services are covered through the plan and aren't paid for under Original Medicare. Most Medicare Advantage Plans offer prescription drug coverage.

Medicare-approved amount - In Original Medicare, this is the amount a doctor or supplier that accepts assignment can be paid. It may be less than the actual amount a doctor or supplier charges. Medicare pays part of this amount and you're responsible for the difference.

Medicare SELECT - A types of Medigap policy that may require you to use hospitals and, in some cases, doctors within its network to be eligible for full benefits.

Medicare prescription drug plan (Part D) - Part D adds prescription drug coverage to Original Medicare, some Medicare Cost Plans, and some Medicare Private-Fee-for-Service Plans, and Medicare Medical Savings Account Plans. These plans are offered by private companies approved by Medicare. Medicare Advantage Plans may also offer prescription drug coverage that follows the same rules as Medicare Prescription Drug Plans.

Medigap - Also known as Medicare supplement. Insurance coverage designed to "fill the gaps" in Original Medicare by paying for certain health care costs not paid for by Medicare.

MSP - Medicare Savings Program. The 4 savings program include; Qualified Medicare Beneficiary Program (QMBS), Special Low-Income Beneficiary Program (SLMBS), Qualifying Individual Program (QIS), and Qualified Disabled and Working Individual Program (QDWI).

O.E.P - Open enrollment period- A six-month period beginning on the first day of the month in which a Medicare beneficiary is both age 65 or older and enrolled in Medicare.

Original Medicare - Part A and Parts B of Medicare.

PACE - Program of All-Inclusive Care for Elderly.

PDP - Prescription drug plan or prescription drug providers.

PFFS - Private fee-for-service.

POS - Point of service plan.

PPO - Preferred provider organizations.

RPPO - Regional preferred provider organizations.

Pre-existing condition - Under a Medigap policy, a condition for which medical treatment or advice was received within six months of the policy's effective date of coverage.

Primary Care Doctor - A doctor who has a primary specialty in family medicine, internal medicine, geriatric medicine, or pediatric medicine; or a nurse practitioner, clinical nurse specialist, or physician assistant.

Referral - A written order from your primary care doctor for you to see a specialist or get certain medical services. In many Health Maintenance Organizations (HMO's), you need to get a referral to see a specialist or to receive medical services, other than emergency care while traveling.

SEP - Special election program.

Service Area - A geographic area where a health insurance plan accepts members if it limits membership based on where people live. For plans that limit membership based on where people live. For plans that limit which doctors and hospitals you may use for (non-emergency) services. The plan may disenroll you if you move out of the plan's service area.

Skilled nursing facility (SNF) care - Skilled nursing care and rehabilitation services provided on a continuous, daily basis, in a skilled nursing facility.

SNP - Special needs plan (the 3 SNP plans include; CSNP, Chronic Care; DSNP, Dual-Eligible; ISNPS, Institutionalized).

State Health Insurance Assistance Program (SHIP)- A state agency that regulates insurance and can provide information about Medigap policies and other private health insurance.

Resources

Centers for Medicare & Medicaid Services
7500 Security Boulevard
Baltimore, Maryland 21244-1850
www.cms.gov

Medicare: 1-800-633-4227. TTY users; 1-877-486-2048, or go to www.medicare.gov.

Social Security: 1-800-772-1213. TTY users; 1-800-325-0778, or www.socialsecurity.gov.

Railroad Benefits (RRB): call 1-800-877-9772. TTY users; 1-312-751-4701.

For retired military; **Department of Defense; Tri-Care for Life (TFL);** 1-866-773-0404. TTY; 1-866-773-0405, or go to tricare.mil/tfl.

Department of Veterans' Affair; 1-800-827-1000. TTY; 1-800-829-4833, or va.gov.

For other information about **Federal employee health benefits. Retirees;** 1-888-767-6738. TTY; 1-800-878-5707: www.opm.gov/healthcare-insurance.

Next is personal information about your Medicare benefits and services at www.mymedicare.gov or Centers for Medicare Services (CMS): www.cms.gov. For Medicaid, www.medicaid.gov.

State Health Assistance Program (SHIP); call 1-800-MEDICARE at 1-800-633-4227 for the local listing in your state.

Additional Medicare publications; visit www.medicare.gov/publications to view, print, or download copies of booklets. Some publications can be ordered and mailed directly to your home. Or you can visit Medicare's Blog at www.blog.medicare.gov.

To compare the quality of plans and providers, you can compare how hospital coverage, how nursing homes compare, how home healthcare companies, dialysis facilities compare, physicians compare, and Medicare plans finders compare. Visit medicare.gov or call your State Health Insurance Assistance Program [SHIP], and the number can be obtained from Medicare by asking for your local SHIP office at 1-800-633-4227. Or, you can visit www.shipcenter.org.

FREE VIDEO TRAINING: You can visit the Author's website @ www.howtonavigatemedicare.com

Book Summary

Now you have a better understanding of Medicare and the various Medicare options that are available to you when you turn 65 or first qualify for Medicare. I wish you the best in selecting a health care plan that will meet your health care needs and fit within your budget.

To help you determine which path you will follow on your Medicare journey, I have included a step-by-step flowchart to help you chart your course through the Medicare Maze.

If you should have any questions, please feel free to contact the author **Michael Kench** at: http://www.howtonavigatemedicare.con

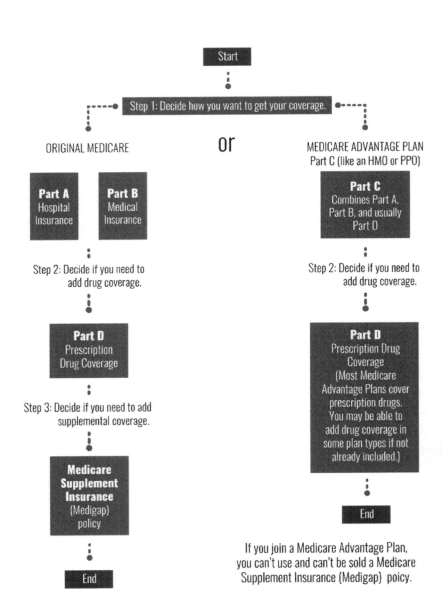

Book Michael Kench to Speak!

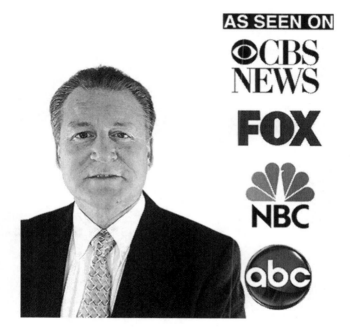

For over two decades, Michael has been educating, entertaining, and helping retirees in the area of Retirement Planning. He covers safe investment strategies during retirement, income planning, 401k rollover options, tax reduction strategies, Social Security & Medicare planning.

His unique style inspires, empowers, and entertains audiences. While giving them the tools and strategies they need to plot a safe and secure course in retirement. He also instructs retirees on how to avoid common financial mistakes most retirees make in retirement.

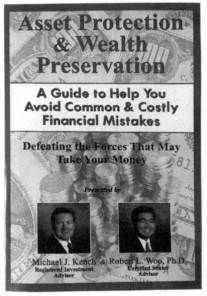

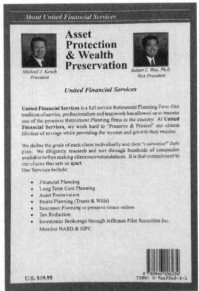

For more info, visit www.howtonavigatemedicare.com or call +1 (714) 386-9808

A Closing Note from Michael J. Kench

As you can probably tell, I love helping individuals with their Retirement Planning.

Retirement planning encompasses several areas and when you retire, there is a major change that occurs. You shift from an Accumulation of assets to a Distribution phase. The way you invest during retirement, IRA, 401K's, Savings, and how you distribute those assets with proper income planning, so that you don't run out-of-money during retirement.

Medicare, Social Security choices, Tax Planning, Estate Planning & Wealth Preservation.

One of the best platforms to ensure that you keep current with Retirement Planning changes and how they impact you during retirement, and to help you avoid common health & financial mistakes in Retirement.

I want to invite you to a <u>Free</u> online and on-demand training course called, **"How to Avoid the Top 10 Most Common Financial Mistakes Retirees Make and Simple Ways to Avoid them."**

This is a complete Step-By-Step training, and it's **FREE**, and you can even ask questions!

Or, you can sign up for my *Free* <u>Newsletter</u> to keep up to date with changes to Medicare! All you have to do is navigate Right Now over to: www.howtonavigatemedicare.com

Made in the USA
Lexington, KY
06 December 2016